THE ESSENTIAL

skin
care
guide

FOR PEOPLE OF COLOUR

THE ESSENTIAL

skin care guide

FOR PEOPLE OF COLOUR

Emade Masango

How To Achieve Healthy and Glowing Skin

For more information, contact the author:
Emade Masango
Email: baesthetics70@gmail.com
Instagram: @embeautyaesthetics

Edited by Bolanle Bodunrin
Cover Design, Formatting, and Layout by Shobola Ibukun

For my children, Gabriella, Jayden, and Kalisha

Acknowledgments

To my husband, my whole world. I thank God every day that I found you; I keep reaching higher and pushing harder, and you give me all the encouragement I need to reach for the stars. You believe in me. Thank you for being the best spouse on earth.

To my daughters and son, Gabriella, Kalisha, and Jayden. I didn't know what it was like to weep with joy until you were born. I am so thankful to be your mother, and I am so proud of you, my little kiddos.

Without you, my parents, I would not have had the education or strength to accomplish any of my goals. Thank you for challenging me so far beyond my comfort zone.

To all the Masango lineage, I am proud to be a member of your bloodline.

A special thanks to Mbamba, Mummy Yeye, and Mummy Teteh for always pushing and encouraging me in all aspects of my life and pushing me to my limits.

Thank you so much, Bolanle, for helping to bring my work to light. You've been a huge help. Even though there were a lot of sleepless nights and stress, our teamwork was incredible.

Thank you for taking the time out of your busy schedule to read my book and for offering feedback, Doctor Gabi. I really appreciate it.

Finally, I would like to thank all of my friends who read my book and offered me honest feedback; you contributed to bringing my book to light.

Table of Contents

Chapter 4

My Skincare Story

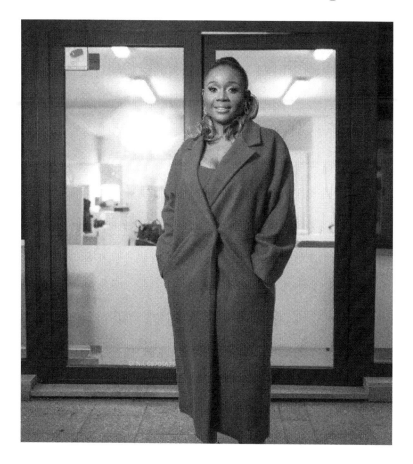

Before having my first child, I did not place much importance on taking care of my skin. Yes, I had a simple regimen of putting body lotion on, but I didn't pay enough attention to my skin. Then, as I was expecting my second child, I developed skin problems and put on weight. I had stretch marks and acne and was chubby and bloated. To cap it all, I experienced hyperpigmentation. My face did not look good at all, and I completely quit socializing. I was devastated.

I wanted a healthy glow on my lovely dark skin. I needed to feel better! I wanted to look good. I had just experienced the incredible event of bringing a kid into the world, for which I was grateful, but I hated my body, which was the very thing that had given my husband and me so much joy in so many ways. Not one to wallow in hopelessness for too long, I acknowledged my wish to feel and look better and started searching for information on how to achieve my aim. I use the word "search" since it is difficult to get enough information on how to care for my particular type of skin. The black skincare sector is, at best, in its infancy when compared to other skin types.

Nevertheless, I persisted in looking until I found the solution. I quickly put my acquired knowledge to use and began making adjustments. I started by watching what I ate more closely, followed by establishing a skincare routine. Additionally, I used affirmations like "Emade, you have beautiful skin," "You are gloriously and wonderfully made," and others when I looked in the mirror. I also worked on losing weight because I had that goal as well. I soon dropped 10 kg (about 22 pounds). My mood improved! My skin also benefited from the weight loss. As the days went by, I became less agitated, irritable, and grumpy. I was overflowing with energy! Even my hubby, bless his heart, began focusing 00more on me, hehe.

I continued for another year to identify my passion after shedding the baby weight, and there it was! My realization that individuals of color like me struggle to keep glowing skin in a region unsuited to our skin type came after spending some time living in Europe. I, at that point, decided I wanted to become an aesthetician! I also wanted to support people in leading healthy lives.

Additionally, as I reflected on my younger years, I realized that my propensity to use my mother's cosmetics without her knowledge hinted at my love for skincare and beauty products. All of these helped me recognize that I had an interest in skincare and beauty even before I became pregnant. I had eczema and dry skin as a child, which had an impact on my self-esteem until I was an adult. Thus, becoming pregnant just brought my passion for skincare to the fore. Who said that negative experiences couldn't lead to positive ones? I had my third child by the time I had started working toward my goal of becoming an aesthetician.

Not long after that, I traveled to London in August 2022 but I returned home with a significant acne breakout. I had a lot going on and didn't pay attention to my diet. I wasn't drinking enough water, and the weather harmed my skin. The truth is that despite all of these excuses, I knew it was my fault for neglecting my skin. I ought to have paid attention.

Your experience as a person of color might resemble mine. You may have a variety of skin problems whether you are pregnant or not, male or female, and you may be wondering what you did to deserve the suffering. Your skin should be radiant and healthy. When you go to social events, you want to look your best. I'm glad to let you know that your worries are over because I'm going to reveal to you tips on how to take care of your skin as a person of color. Your skin colour could be a brilliant fair, burnished brown, or even a lustrous dark. It could be dry, normal, oily, and everything in between. In and out of season, in and out of Africa, I have got you covered.

To start with, I have revealed in this book common skin diseases that plague people of color so that you can recognise them. Naturally, this is followed by advice on the best items to use for each disease, product suggestions, and a straightforward skincare routine that is appropriate for your skin type, age, and season of the year. Finally, I provided lifestyle advice for maintaining healthy, glowing skin. With these fantastic insights, your skin will "give radiant" all year long.

Say "yes!" if you're prepared to have your skin look its best. Let's do this!

01

A Tale of Acne, Pimples
and Stubborn Blackheads

My skin was smooth and fair before I moved to Europe until the environment shift, the weather, getting older, and my eating habits messed it all up. I started to develop acne and hyperpigmentation. It was a nightmare. I was so embarrassed that I avoided going out and having fun with friends and family. It was at this point I discovered skin types.

Skin Type

There are four main categories of skin types that we are all born with regardless of our race: normal skin, combination skin, oily skin, and dry skin.[1]

Dry Skin

Natural oil (sebum) production on this type of skin is insufficient. Research has found that because black skin cannot contain enough water, its top layer does not stay moisturized for very long, leaving it dry and flaky. If you have dry skin, you'll find that makeup doesn't adhere to your face well without going spotty after a while.

---

1   (Yowell, n.d.)

Also, keep in mind that dry skin may be a skin disorder due to environmental factors that cause skin dehydration.

Oily Skin

If your pores create too many natural oils, you have oily skin. In this instance, your skin tends to be oily, glossy, rough, and thick. It also tends to attract blackheads. If you have oily skin, resist the urge to apply harsh products to it because the results will not be pleasant.

Combination Skin

As it is difficult to discover people with skin types that can easily fall into a specific category, this is the most typical skin type. Your skin may have oily patches here and dry patches there. You can have the infamous T-zone, where your cheeks and temples are dry yet your forehead and nose are greasy.

Normal Skin

The proper amount of perspiration and sebum is present on normal skin. Smooth texture and modestly sized pores that are visible on the skin's surface balance it out. Sadly, only a small number of people have this classic skin type.

The Uniqueness of the Black Skin

All races share the same basic skin structure, but the distinctiveness of black skin is due to the presence of melanin. People of color secrete a lot of melanin in their skin, which is not a coincidence given that we have historically lived in places with a higher distribution of ultraviolet light (UVR). For instance, regions like Africa are close to the equator.

There are also many different shades of black skin in Africa. Depending on how close they are to the equator, some are rich dark, dark, chocolate, brown, fair, somewhat fair, excessively fair, and so on. However, melanin, a chemical that is lacking in the skin, is what unites all of these skin tones.

Leslie Baumann's Skin Types

Dermatologist, Dr. Leslie Baumann,[2] also found more skin types that are distinct from the ones already discussed. She kept the pigmented or non-pigmented (P/N), wrinkled or unwrinkled (W/T), and dry or oily skin types (D/O) categories. The sensitive skin type is another option (S).

This additional classification is crucial because it enables us to correctly assess our skin type and choose the appropriate solutions to treat it. This classification's inclusion and identification of dark-skinned people is noteworthy because they frequently have the PT and DS skin types, which make them more reactive to certain skin care regimens (more on this in chapter 4) and susceptible to specific skin conditions/problems.[3]

With this knowledge in hand, let's look at some of the prevalent skin disorders and conditions that affect people of color below.

Common Skin Conditions in People of Colour

As previously noted, persons of color are more likely to experience particular skin disorders. This may be the result of elements like certain weather conditions, pollution, food, using the incorrect products for your skin type, and so forth. To name a few of them:

---

2   (Oliveira, n.d.)

3   (Obafemi Awolowo University, Ladoke Akintola University of Technology, and Otike-Odibi 2019)

Acnes

Other names for them include zits, blackheads, and whiteheads. People frequently ask me if acne and pimples are the same. No, and yes. I'll explain. A skin condition that results in pimples is acne. A pimple is a tiny swelling on the face that develops when oil, dead skin cells, germs, and dirt clog the pores of your skin, which are typically found on your face, back, chest, or shoulders. On the other side, one can be called to have acne if they frequently get pimples. Acne is a common problem for individuals of color.

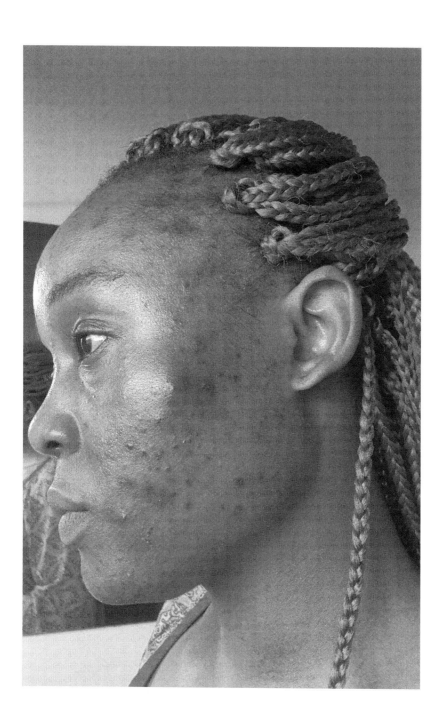

According to a study,[4] sebum production is the reason why persons of color (African Americans and Hispanics) are more likely to have clinical acne. We see this effect more strongly in temperate regions like Europe where our skin is prone to produce extra oil to combat dehydration. In an actual sense, sebum is an "oily, waxy substance produced by your body's sebaceous glands."[5] According to a piece by the Harvard Medical School,[6] sebum contains "a complex mixture of fatty acids, sugars, waxes, and other natural chemicals that form a protective barrier against water evaporation". These sebaceous glands are found all over our body except for the palms and the soles of our feet. Our faces have the most sebaceous glands totaling about 900 in number.[7]

Due to its difficulty adapting to stress, pollution, hard water, severe humidity, excessive wind, and a lack of sunlight, black skin produces too much sebum under these circumstances. Acne and hyperpigmentation result when dead skin cells, perspiration, dust, and other items floating in the air are combined (I will be getting to this in a minute). Don't pop that zit just yet—these are the potential reasons for that small bulge that's strewn across your face and is making you so angry— not before allowing it to turn red and not after wiping your hands on a tissue before popping it; else, hyperpigmentation will result.

---

4   (Kimball, n.d.)
5   (Cobb, Pedroja, and Ramachandran 2020)
6   ("Dry Skin" 2019)
7   (Smith and Thiboutot 2008)

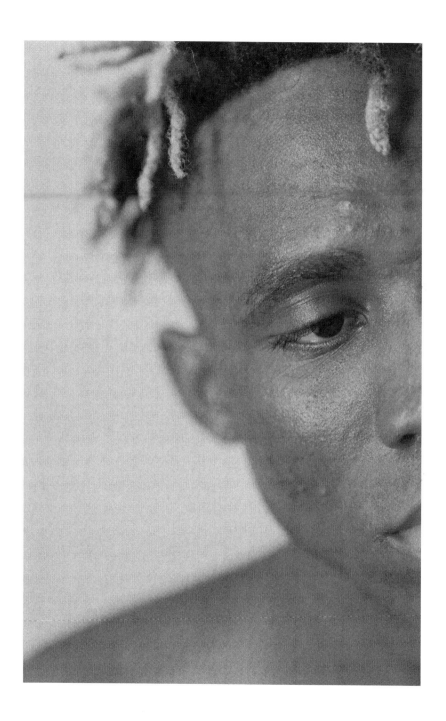

Hyperpigmentation

Do you know about the black mark on your face that emerges when a pimple "heals"? We call it hyperpigmentation. If you pop your pimple with your bare hands, or if your pimple-popping friend assists you to do so with her bare hands, you will get acne scars or post-inflammatory hyperpigmentation (PIH). After their skin has undergone acne-related stress, such as scarring, darker skin types get PIH more frequently than other skin types. The skin darkens as the wound closes, and it will take an agonizingly long time for the color to return to normal.

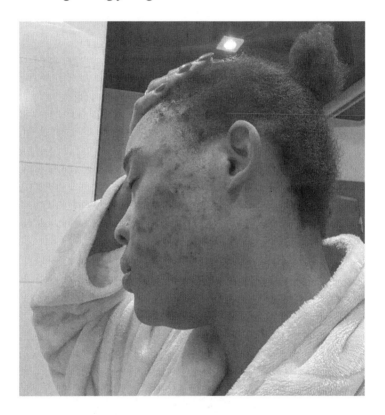

Other factors can contribute to hyperpigmentation in people with black skin. Black skin types have more melanin than other skin types, making us more susceptible to hyperpigmentation in certain circumstances. Other than acne, eczema, and melasma (more on this soon), infections from rashes, insect bites, scrapes, burns, lupus, and several cosmetic treatments are among the causes of hyperpigmentation.

Do you want to know how hyperpigmentation appears on your skin? Hyperpigmentation can appear in a variety of colors depending on the cause and your type of black skin. Therefore, keep an eye out for any tan, brown, dark brown, grey-brown, blue-grey, purple, or black spots or patches on your skin. Be wary of any areas that appear darker than the surrounding region in general.

Even though it is safe, it stays in our skin for a long time and can have negative psychological effects in addition to causing emotional anguish. If you are bothered by it, get it thoroughly. Depending on its etiology and as recommended by your dermatologist, there are various techniques to cure hyperpigmentation. Some treatments include applying sunscreen (see chapter 2 for additional details), staying away from skin-irritating cosmetics, taking prescription medications for conditions like lupus, and getting help for acne and eczema.

Melasma

When persons of color are overexposed to sunshine, they develop this type of hyperpigmentation. If you have melasma, you may notice dark patches on your face and other regions of your body, depending on the color of your skin. It happens when our skin's melanocytes create an excessive amount of pigment. It is important to highlight that individuals with dark complexion (black or brown) have more melanocytes than individuals of lighter skin. The skin cells that make melanin are called melanocytes.

Additionally, according to data, melasma tends to develop in adults rather than children, more frequently in the 20s, 30s, or 40s, and less frequently in men (less than 10%). Sun exposure, hormonal changes during pregnancy or the use of birth control, exposure to active chemicals in some skincare products, and extreme sun exposure are some other reasons for melasma.

Melasma can appear on the cheeks, nose, forehead, upper lip, and chin, among other parts of our bodies. Additionally, you may see discoloration or dark patches on the arms, chest, shoulder, and neck. The patches can appear in a variety of patterns, including blotchy, solid, freckle-like, and irregular.

It is not hazardous, like certain skincare disorders, but it can be rather uncomfortable and unsightly to the eyes. You might discover that you avoid social situations. The good news is that it is quickly diagnosed and effectively treated. Sometimes it simply affects the skin's surface, but it can also penetrate well beneath the skin's surface.

You should stay out of the sun's direct rays to prevent melasma. So on sunny days, use caps or apply skin protection products like sunscreen (see Chapter 2 guidelines). A healthy weight and proper diet are also beneficial for your skin in general. You should also address underlying medical conditions that lead to hormone imbalances that may promote melasma. Among these include thyroid disease and prostate, menopause, and low testosterone, among others.

Razor Bumps

It is also known as pseudofolliculitis barbae.[8] Let's just call it "razor bumps" since that's not too long a name. Among men of color, this skin conduction is fairly prevalent. When curly hair grows back into the skin after shaving, it affects the beard area. Ingrown hair is the term for this hair. Shaving sharpens the hairs in the beard, which subsequently curve into the skin and cause inflammation, lumps, or scars that resemble keloid growths.

Let your beard grow like a mountain man's (I'm kidding) to avoid razor rashes. However, if you want a more subdued appearance, you can use a barber clipper after moistening the region with shaving cream, gel, or powder. This assists in avoiding the discomfort and friction that lead to ingrown hairs. Additionally, avoid shaving a region too tightly or frequently. If you currently have razor bumps, wait until they have all completely healed before shaving again.

Ashy Skin

How many times have you heard a girlfriend jokingly tell her other black girlfriends to "go on with your ashy self!"? It's funny but not so funny because ashiness sucks! Every race experiences ashy skin but people of colour experience it more. Our skin becomes dry, flaky, and grey. Not a good look at all. So no to ashiness!

Dermatosis papulosa Nigra

Probably without realizing it, you have seen Dermatosis Papulosa Nigra on other people's faces. You might even possess it. Skin tags or peduncles are other names for it. Do you now recognize it? Small,

---

8   (Ollennu 2021)

short black or brown lumps on the face or neck are its defining feature. Dermatosis papulosa nigra is that little protruding stump in the face that you want to pull out or wonder how it got there in the first place!

It is frequently observed in people with black complexion, is regarded as harmless, and usually begins during puberty. As one age, they may increase in number. Even while skin tags aren't harmful, some of us choose to have them removed, which is possible with laser surgery and other procedures.

Vitiligo

All races are impacted by this uncommon skin ailment, although black skin shows it the most. When this happens, lighter patches of skin start to appear on the skin. Vitiligo is caused, in scientific words, by the death of melanocytes in the skin.

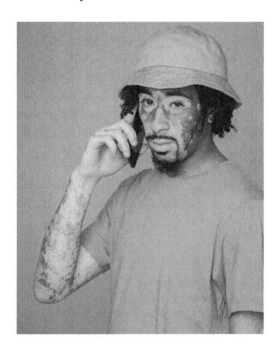

The face—mouth, nose, eyes, and head—as well as other sun-exposed regions of the body—are where vitiligo typically first appears. People with vitiligo frequently face stigmatization and discrimination. Although it is difficult to predict whether someone may have vitiligo, it frequently starts before the age of 40. Currently, there is no treatment for the skin disease, however, it is recommended that sunscreen be used to prevent any skin-related problems from arising in general.

Keloids

This type of raised scar develops following the healing of a skin injury. Puncture wounds, cuts, tattoos, piercings, severe acne, insect bites, chickenpox surgery scars, injection sites, tightly braided hair, shaving, and other skin conditions can all result in keloids.

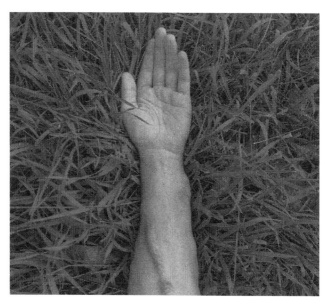

After healing is complete, scar tissue doesn't stop developing; instead, it keeps doing so and can occasionally become very enormous. Although it hasn't been proven, scientists argue that keloid development happens when the body overproduces collagen in reaction to damage. The majority of black and brown people have keloids. Although they may first appear red, they eventually become darker than a person's skin.

Pityriasis Alba

Children and teenagers are affected by this skin disorder. Scales of oblong or circular hypopigmented lesions are how it manifests. It resembles eczema and atopic dermatitis. Its genesis is a mystery.

And that brings us to the end of the most prevalent skin issues affecting persons of color. Let's look at several things we may use to either completely shield our skin from them or to treat them. So let's go!

02

Of Cleansers, Toners,
Serums, and Moisturisers

etting items that are suitable for black skin should be our main priority. Many of the skincare items we can buy at the grocery store cannot fully benefit our skin. As a result, we are forced to manage the ones we can, hoping that they will be useful to us. Additionally, many dermatologists and aestheticians don't spend enough time learning about black skin. To make matters worse, I've seen that, except for individuals in the entertainment and music industries, people of color tend to underestimate the value of caring for their skin. We prefer to purchase solitary products to see the effects right away rather than a skincare package for total body care. We must stop now!

The truth is that skin care involves much more than just slathering on some body lotion. Additionally, you need to utilize skincare products carefully because some of them have harsh components that might harm your skin. Therefore, I will discuss the main types of skin care products in this chapter and then offer suggestions for ingredients you must have in your skincare products. I can't wait to share them with you! Continue reading if you are as excited as I am, and get ready to go shopping thereafter!

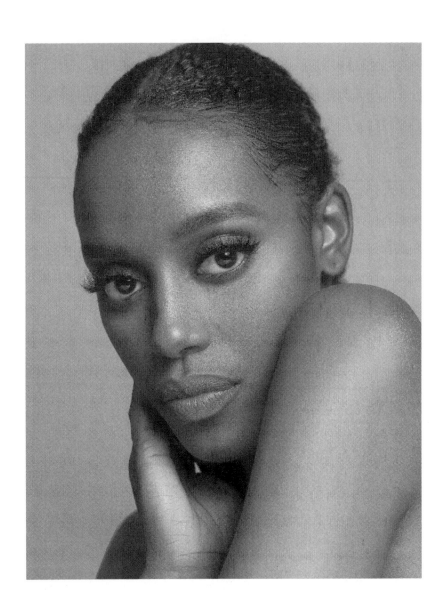

The Essential Skin Care Guide For People of Colour

Must-Have Skincare Products with the Right Components For People of Colour[9]

Cleanser

It is recommended that we wash our faces twice a day to remove bacteria, sweat, dirt, and makeup. You must get your skin type diagnosed o get the proper cleanser for your face and avoid using one that is inappropriate for you.

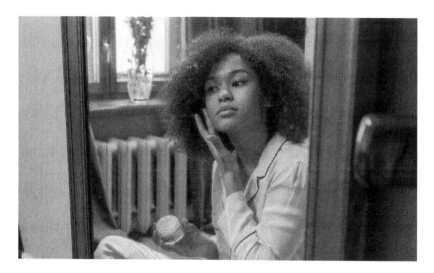

With a few notable exceptions, people of color typically have oily skin and acne, thus a gel cleanser would be the ideal choice. It is gel-like, as the name would imply, and works well to unclog pores clogged with excess sebum and sweat. These kinds of cleansers are ideal for thorough cleaning.

Your gel cleanser should contain:

- Niacinamide (controls sebum)
- Salicylic acid (unclogs pores)

---

9   (Racho, n.d.)

- Glycerin (hydrates skin)
- D panthenol (anti-inflammatory)
- Acne calm (Anti-bacterial complex)

Product Recommendations: iS Clinical Cleansing Complex (All Skin Types), First Aid Beauty Face Cleanser (Dry Skin & Sensitive Skin), Keep the Peace Cleanser by Versed (Acne-prone Skin)[10]

Toner

Shrinks pores and returns skin's normal pH, which may have been affected by soaps, excessive oil production, or even chemicals in cleansers, and is typically used after a cleanser. To remove extra makeup or other traces on the face, use it twice a day.

Your toner should typically contain:
- salicylic acid like lactic, glycolic, malic, or beta-hydroxy acids (takes care of large pores and boosts collagen production)
- Niacinamide, vitamin B3 (Acne & Oily Skin)
- amino acids, ceramides, hyaluronic acid, fatty acids, triglycerides, phospholipids, linoleic acid, glycerin (dry/ mature skin)

If you have sensitive skin, look for a toner without alcohol. Please be aware that toners, like other skin care products, are used to treat various skin conditions, so choose the proper one for your skin type or concerns. In the end, you might need to seek the advice of a dermatologist for the right testing. If you are already aware of your skin type, consult an aesthetician.

---

10   (Mitchell, n.d.)

Product Recommendations: Obagi Medical Nu-Derm Toner (All Skin Types), Rose Deep Hydration Facial Toner (Dry Skin), Burt's Bees Sensitive Toner With Aloe Vera (Sensitive Skin)

Serums

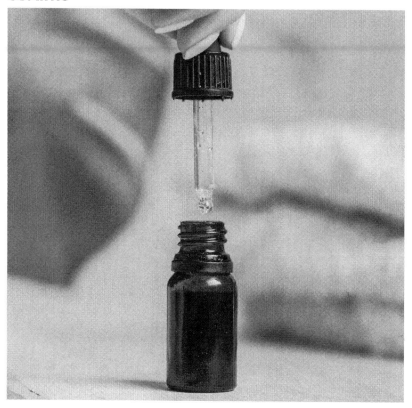

Because of its lighter texture than moisturizers, this incredible skin care product deeply moisturizes your skin. Antioxidants in it can help prevent skin damage. Additionally, it contains anti-aging ingredients like retinoids and peptides that promote the formation of collagen. It works best when applied after washing your face, but you may also use it before moisturizing.

Face serums are adaptable and can be mixed with moisturizers, face creams, and masks to treat various skin issues in-depth, such as hyperpigmentation, dry skin, wrinkles, sagging skin, and fine lines.[11]

Typically, you can look out for the following ingredients in your serums:

- Retinol, antioxidants, peptides, and stem cells (anti-aging)
- Sodium hyaluronate and glutamine (for firmness)
- Vitamin C, arbutin, kojic acid, liquorice extract, and alpha hydroxy acids (hyperpigmentation)
- Hyaluronic acid, essential fatty acids, ceramides, and niacinamide (for hydration)
- Herbal extracts, chamomile, aloe, and calendula (Redness of skin)
- Lactic acid, liquorice, lemongrass, and aloe vera (dark spots and large spots)

Product Recommendations: Murad Retinol Youth Renewal Serum (fights fine lines and wrinkles), Neocutis Bio Serum Firm (collagen boosting), PCA Skin Hyaluronic Acid Boosting Serum (For dry skin).

Moisturiser

This is yet another crucial skincare item that belongs in your pack. Finding the appropriate types for your gorgeous skin tone might be difficult with so many options available in stores, but don't worry— I'm here to assist. You still need the additional layer of protection that

---

11   (Quinn, n.d.)

a moisturizer provides, even if the sebum and perspiration on your skin are in the proper proportion. Although oily skin may not require as much moisturizing as other skin types.

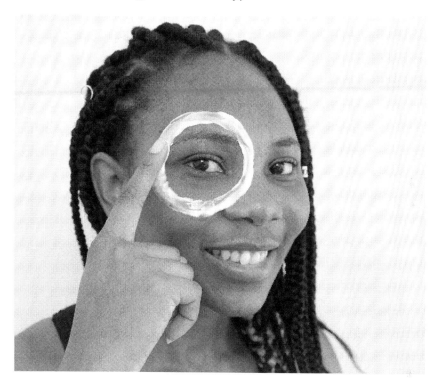

Generally speaking, a cream moisturizer is preferable for someone with dry skin. If oily, check your moisturizer for "non-comedogenic" components. To find the best products for you if you have sensitive skin, schedule a patch test appointment with a dermatologist.

Get moisturizers for combination skin that will regulate your oily patches while also keeping your dry patches moistened. If you are older, your moisturizer should have anti-aging compounds such as vitamins A, B, C, D, and E that promote collagen production in the skin.

People of color frequently have combination skin, dry skin, or both, so essential components like ceramides, glycerin, and/or hyaluronic acid should be present in our moisturizers. [12] Gel moisturizers are generally safe for all skin types on persons of color when they include the correct components.

Your morning (AM) gel moisturiser should essentially contain:
- Niacinamide 2% (controls sebum)
- Vitamin C (sodium ascorbyl phosphate) 2%
- D panthenol, Allantoin, Green tea extract arnica (anti-inflammatory)
- Glycerin 3% (hydrator)
- AcneCalm (antibacterial complex)

Your evening (PM)) gel moisturiser should essentially contain:
- Alpha Arbutin (anti-pigmentation)
- Vitamin C (sodium ascorbyl phosphate) (brightening)
- Allantoin (Anti-inflammatory)
- Niacinamide (sebum control)
- Glycerin (hydrating)
- Salicylic acid (unclogs pores)
- Retinol 0.1% (increases cell turnover)
- Tetrahexyldecyl ascorbate (Stimulates collagen)
- Retinaldehyde 0.1% (increases cell turnover)
- AcneCalm (anti-bacterial complex)
- Ferulic acid (antioxidant)
- Green tea extract (anti-inflammatory)
- Ceramides (skin restoring)

---

12 ("The Best Moisturizers for Your Skin Type", n.d.)

The Essential Skin Care Guide For People of Colour

And you are good to go!

Product Recommendations: SkinMedica Rejuvenative Moisturizer (for normal skin), Epionce Intensive Nourishing Cream (for dry skin), La Roche-Posay Effaclar Mat Daily Moisturizer for Oily Skin (for oily skin)[13]

Sunscreen

This lotion shields your skin from UV deterioration year-round. If you live in a warmer climate and are a person of color, you should take sunscreen use even more seriously. The use of sunscreen is recommended by experts every day, not just on the beach but even in cool climes and during daily runs.

A minimum SPF of 30 is recommended for sunscreen, or 50 if you plan to spend a lot of time outside. For best protection, reapply your sunscreen at least every two hours. Choose a lightweight, greasy-free sunscreen if your skin is oily.

- Niacinamide (Acne-prone skin)
- Turmeric (sensitive skin)
- Vitamin C (oily skin)
- SPF 30, hyaluronic acid, Vitamins C and E, Green tea extract (dry skin)
- Probiotic extracts, pineapple, papaya, butterfly ginger roots (combination skin)
- Tranexamic acid, Niacinamide, Phenylethyl resorcinol, Glycerin, Reflective Mica (To fight Hyperpigmentation)
- SPF 50, Peptides, Glucosamine HCL (Anti-aging)

---

13   ("15 Best Moisturizers For Black Skin In 2022 (Face & Body)" 2022)

Product Recommendations: Obagi Sun Shield Matte Broad Spectrum SPF 50 (Oily Skin), Sunday Riley Light Hearted Broad Spectrum SPF 30 Sunscreen (Sensitive Skin), Neocutis Journée Revitalizing Day Cream SPF 30 (Dry Skin)

Exfoliator

This skincare item is intended to remove dead skin cells from your skin, leaving it smooth, young-looking, and fresh, like the skin of a newborn. Physical or chemical exfoliators are both used. While a chemical exfoliant dissolves and sheds away dead skin cells, physical exfoliator chips away at them on the face until they are all gone. Please note that it is not always necessary to exfoliate dry skin.

Your exfoliator should contain:

- Glycerin 5% (water magnet)
- Salicylic acid 2% (unclogs pores, for acne-prone skin)
- Green tea extract and sage (to soothe)

Product Recommendations: Alpyn Beauty Creamy Cleanser with Fruit Enzyme and AHA (fights acne), Jan Marini Skin Zyme (Smoother Skin), Fenty Beauty Total Cleans'r (Deep Cleansing).

Treatment

These are products that are used to treat particular skin issues like hyperpigmentation, acne, dark spots, inflammation, wrinkles, and more. They can be found in a variety of forms, including serums, lotions, face gels, pads for the face, solutions, and more. As soon as you notice a skin condition, make sure to treat it until it entirely disappears; if not, consult a physician or aesthetician.

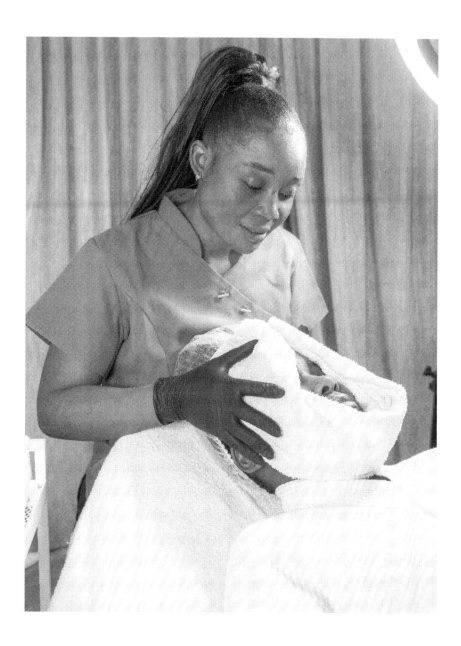

Active ingredients in treatments include:

- Tretinoin, adapalene (fine lines and wrinkles)
- Salicylic acid, benzoyl peroxide (acne)
- Vitamin C (anti-aging)

Oils

No matter your skin type, you may consider using facial oils enriched with nutrients because they assist in making your skin resilient. For improved results, you may also incorporate a few drops of it into your serums or moisturizers. Please note that not all oils are good for your skin. Be wary of fragrant oils because they can increase skin sensitivity. Your best bet for oils is non-fragrant plant oils.

Oils to look out for include:
- Tea tree oil, Jojoba (for acne-prone skin)
- Argan Oil, Vitamin E (anti-aging)
- Olive, Sunflower, Barrage Seed Oil (dry skin)
- Vitamin E, yangu, argan (sensitive skin)

Product Recommendations: Eminence Rosehip Triple C+E Firming Oil (anti-ageing), Herbivore Botanicals Orchid Facial Oil (Acne-prone Skin)

Chemical Peel

This product is more effective at removing excess dead skin cells than exfoliators. They peel off the skin's outer layer and are used for skin treatments. You can peel once in two weeks but not too often. They are effective in addressing acne, wrinkles, fine lines, and hyperpigmentation. If you want to do a chemical peel, it is best to consult with a professional dermatologist or aesthetician to avoid using products that are not appropriate for your skin and thus damage it.

Active ingredients in your product include glycolic, salicylic, or lactic acids. Your product should contain any of these ingredients.

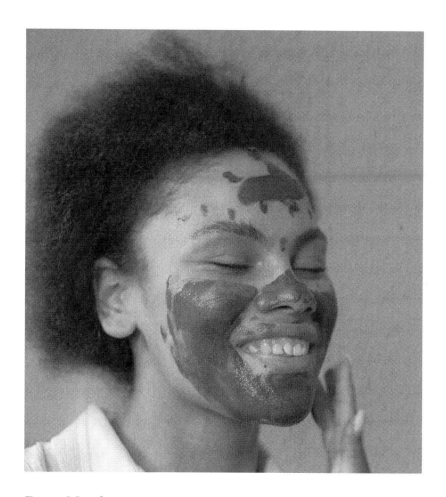

Face Mask

Face masks are a great product for all skin types evidenced by the varieties available on the market. Face masks can be drying, brightening, or even moisturizing.

Active ingredients in face masks include:
- Green tea, allantoin (damage repairing & skin softening)
- Lactic acid (exfoliant)
- Kaolin clay (Deep cleansing)
- Coenzyme q10, Alpha lipoic acid (skin healing)

- Aloe vera (calming effect)
- Cucumber (toning)
- Bilberry extract (skin rejuvenation)
- Vitamin E (prevents dryness)

Product Recommendations: Natura Bissé Essential Shock Intense Mask (damage repair), NeoStrata Glycolic Microdermabrasion Polish (for smooth and professional finish)

Eye Cream

Finally, there are skin care items designed exclusively for the eye area. They deal with problems like crow's feet, sagginess, and dark circles. To put it mildly, the skin around our eyes is a telltale sign of exhaustion, aging, sun damage, and lack of sleep.

Ingredients to look out for in your eye creams:
- Retinol, peptide (collagen stimulation)
- Arnica, vitamin K, caffeine, niacinamide (minimize puffiness and dark circles)
- Hyaluronic acid, Viti's flower stem cell, omega fatty acids (for dark circles)
- Argan oil, avocado oil, coconut oil (for wrinkles, crow feet)
- Vitamin C, peptides, black cumin seed oil (eye bags)
- Flavonoids, blueberry extract, pro xylane (anti-aging)
- Green tea, aloe vera, chamomile, liquorice root (sensitive skin)

Product Recommendations: SkinMedica Instant Bright Eye Cream (for firmness and hydration), Paula's Choice Omega+ Complex Eye Cream (for tired-looking eyes), HydroPeptide Eye Authority (anti-aging eye cream)

Whew! Who said the industry of skincare wasn't serious? Finally, these are the skin care products that ought to always be in your skincare kit. The following chapter is where you should go if you want to learn how to use your products.

03

Rub, Spray, Shine
& Glow All Your Life

If you read Chapter 2 carefully, you will understand that choosing the correct products and understanding how to use them are the keys to establishing an effective skin routine. You won't achieve the results you want as a person of color if your skincare routine consists of simply spreading lotion or cream all over your body. It's noteworthy to note that as you get older, your skincare routine gradually adjusts. In your 40s, what worked in your 20s might not. Therefore, pay close attention to what I have to say to you in this chapter.

What kind of skincare routine, in general, is effective for skin of any color or type?

Here's a simple formula:
C+T+S+M+S= Glowing Skin

In other words, wash your face with warm water after taking a bath, then begin using your cleanser. Depending on the kind you use (gel or liquid), dab a blob on your face and rub it around in a circular motion to remove any debris and toxins that your soap was unable to remove. With warm water, rinse. Apply a fresh cloth to your face. Apply a <u>toner</u> next and massage it all over your face. Follow up by applying your <u>serum</u> to your face to make you look younger. Apply your <u>moisturizer</u> next to regulate oil production, keep your skin firm and hydrated, and finish with your <u>sunscreen</u> to protect your skin. It should be applied 30 minutes before heading outside.

Skin Care Secrets for All Ages

I had zero interest in skincare when I was in my 20s. It was uncommon for my skin to act up, so I didn't pay attention to it. Washing my face every night wasn't even on the table because I hardly ever wore makeup. As for me, I skipped sunscreen. However, as I approached my 30th birthday, I saw a few lines and wrinkles on my face! I began to pay attention, you better believe it.

Isn't this a person of color's typical skin care story? Until something goes wrong, we get married or start a relationship and want to impress our significant other, ladies rarely give skin care any thought. On the other hand, good skin comes easily to certain people, and they rarely take care of it. I had no idea how important SPF50 (sunscreen) was until I started getting breakouts and had skin issues.

All I'm trying to say is that you shouldn't wait till you have skin problems to start caring for your skin. Use the knowledge in this book, which contains all the details you require to begin a skincare routine. Your skin is a vital component of your body. It is your largest and most adaptable organ. Your entire well-being is impacted if something were to happen to it. Therefore, always take care of it! Now, let's talk about how to maintain healthy skin for the rest of your life.

Pre-Teens to Teenage years

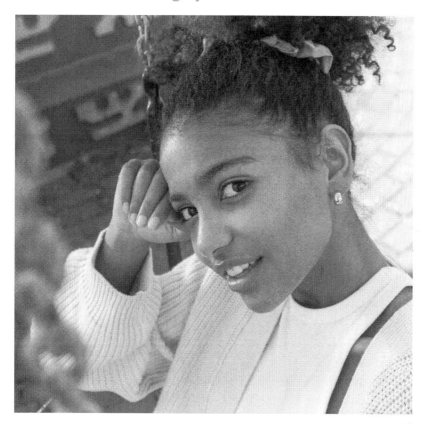

Puberty is a stage of life that you are going through in this season. You might start getting acne and other skin conditions at this age. Additionally, your skin can start to produce too much oil. If you have oily skin or are in your teenage years, follow these skin care guidelines:

In the morning (AM Routine)

- Use a gel cleanser or gentle face wash to unclog your pores
- Apply a non-comedogenic moisturiser (no fragrance!)
- Round off with a non-comedogenic sunscreen

In the evening (PM Routine)
- Use a salicylic acid face wash to clear out pores
- Use a 2-5% niacinamide serum
- Round off with a non-comedogenic moisturiser

To treat acne:

Instead of using a salicylic acid wash to cure acne, use a benzoyl peroxide wash and wash it off after one minute. Use it on your face no more than twice a month to avoid overusing it and risking irritation or flaking. Change to a salicylic acid leave-on toner if you don't see any improvement, and add azelaic acid if you start to see red markings.

To treat a pimple:

Apply a salicylic acid wash, then a salicylic acid toner, and then cover the pimple with a hydrocolloid patch overnight to allow it to absorb extra sebum production. To prevent skin thinning due to a negative side effect, avoid using steroid creams for an extended period. Consult your doctor right away if skin issues worsen.[14]

---

14   (Rattan 2022)

When You Turn 20

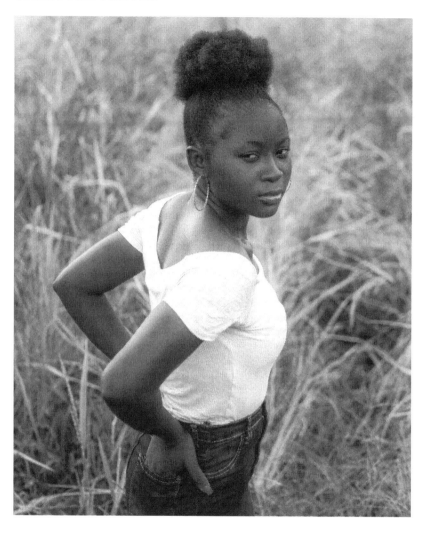

I advise you to take more photos than ever because your skin is the most lovely at this point, haha. Your skin is popping, to use a slang term, because your collagen and elastin are at their peak! However, beyond the age of 21, you lose 1% of your collagen annually, and by your mid-twenties, your body is producing less collagen and elastin.

By your late 20s, hormonal abnormalities that might cause breakouts are more likely to occur. So, in your 20s, I advise you to start using skin care products containing Vitamin A and Retinol. Use SPF50 as well to delay aging. To treat breakouts, you should have your salicylic acid wash nearby.

AM Routine
- Cleanse
- Moisturise
- Apply SPF50

PM Routine
- Double cleanse to remove makeup (if applicable) and sunscreen
- Use salicylic acid wash if you have acne
- Moisturise (use gel moisturiser with Vitamin A for oily skin and to prevent aging)

When You Turn 30

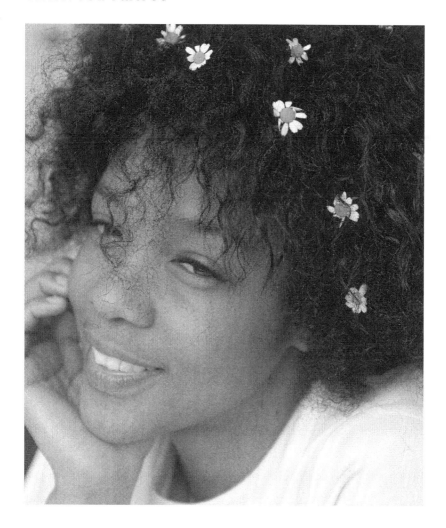

When you reach the age of 30, your skin will start to show specific characteristics, such as dark spots, wrinkles, fine lines, crowfeet, hardness, and so forth. There's no need to worry; you are simply aging. Your skincare regimen must now be updated.

Aging, which is brought on by a decline in collagen formation and a slower rate of cell turnover, is the main issue you have to deal with after you are past your twenties. To stop the accumulation of UV damage, you must also shield your skin from the sun.

Make sure your products have the following elements if you want to have beautiful, healthy skin in your 30s and beyond:

- Retinol
- Hyaluronic acid
- Vitamin C
- Vitamin A
- SPF 50 every two hours for protection from the sun

AM Routine

- Cleanse
- Moisturise with non-fragranced moisturiser
- Apply SPF50 and wear anti-melasma sunglasses and a wide-brimmed hat when going out in the sun

PM Routine

- Double cleanse to remove makeup and sunscreen
- Apply toner with humectants for skin hydration
- Exfoliate 1-2 times every week to remove dead cells
- Apply tyrosinase inhibitors
- Moisturise for added hydration

Lifestyle changes include:

- Using the right products for your skin type
- Exfoliating regularly to do away with dead cells which easily accumulate as you grow older
- Pay attention to your chest and neck! They are also delicate

parts of your body

- Use eye creams
- Adopt a healthy diet such as consuming lots of fruits, vegetables, and water
- Remove your makeup before going to bed to prevent clogged pores and breakouts.
- Use roller jades. They help increase blood circulation thereby encouraging collagen production.

Finally, remember the formula I shared with you earlier, as you enter your 30s, it will change to:

C+E+T+S+EC+M+S= Glowing Skin, E being Exfoliator and EC being Eye Cream

Take note!

When You Turn 40

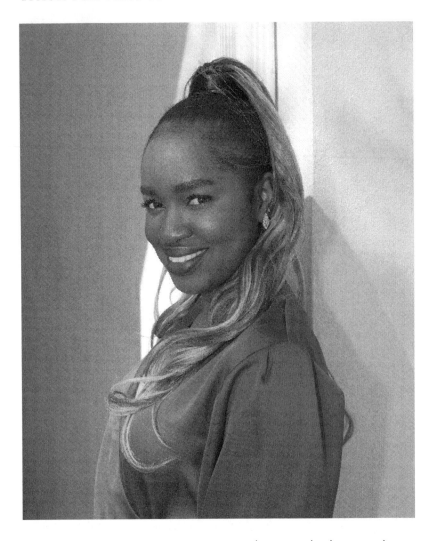

Your body may experience more hormonal changes in your forties, such as a reduction in the production of oestrogen and glycosaminoglycan. And your skin will respond in unison—becoming drier, duller, and more wrinkled, with larger pores and increased hyperpigmentation. You might also notice a lack of skin elasticity, which can result in wrinkles and loose skin. Melasma may get worse if you've been exposed to UV radiation a lot. So how can you properly take care of your skin in your 40s? The following ingredients are required for your products:

- Hyaluronic acid, urea, and glycerin (to strengthen the skin barrier)
- Vitamin A, Peptides, Fat-soluble Vitamin C (to stimulate collagen production)
- SPF 50 and Tyrosinase inhibitors at nighttime (for sun protection)

AM Routine

- Cleanse
- Apply a fattier moisturiser with hyaluronic acid
- Use SPF50 every two hours

PM Routine

- Double cleanse
- Use hyaluronic acid for toning
- Exfoliate at least two nights by week
- Avoid using harsh scrubs
- On nights when you are not exfoliating, apply retinol, and moisturize with a combination of vitamin c, peptides, and Tyrosinase inhibitors.

Lifestyle changes:

- Wear wide-brimmed hats for sun protection
- Use tyrosinase inhibitors at night

When You Turn 50 and Older

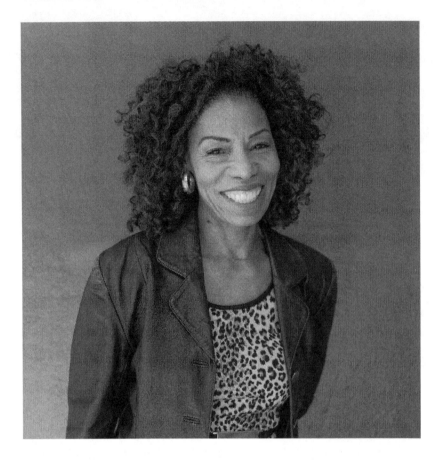

Your skin is producing less collagen at the cellular level, which results in loose skin. Your pores are also more noticeable, and your cell turnover is slower, resulting in dull skin. Additionally, environmental variables may cause your skin to become dryer, your eye wrinkles to deepen, and your skin to become irritated. Ingredients necessary are:

- Vitamin A & Fat-soluble Vitamin C (for loose skin and dull skin)
- Fatty acids like Omega 3, hyaluronic acid, ceramides, and niacinamide (to fight dry skin and wrinkles)
- Aloe and Green Tea (to fight inflammation)

The Essential Skin Care Guide For People of Colour

AM Routine
- Cleanse with a gel wash
- Moisturise with fatty moisturiser and hyaluronic acid
- Apply SPF50 fortified with antioxidant

PM Routine
- Double cleanse to remove makeup and sunscreen
- Use a toner with niacinamide, hyaluronic acid
- Exfoliate with a hydrating chemical exfoliant like lactic acid
- Use active ingredients in your moisturiser like ceramides, peptides, and squalene.

Now let's talk about how to take care of your skin in different seasons.

All-Seasons Skincare Secrets for People of Colour

Apart from a skincare regime, in different seasons, your skin needs a different kind of attention and I'll show you what to do in a jiffy.

Summer Skincare Secrets

The season is hot and sticky. We are going to the beach and spending more time in the sun, but we still need to stay away from the ashiness! So how can we make summer days more pleasant for our melanin-rich skin? Keep up your skincare routine! You must use your cleanser and moisturizer if you want to control sebum production. Additionally, you should exfoliate frequently. Last but not least, remember your SPF for sun protection.

Fall & Winter Skincare Secrets

Because there is less moisture in the air and because there are naturally fewer ceramides and water molecules in the skin, black skin is more vulnerable to dehydration and dryness in colder climates. To protect your skin in the winter:

- Drink more water to stay hydrated
- Eat proteins food for skin elasticity
- Incorporate Omega 3 (fatty acids) into your diet. You can look for similar foods e.g flax seeds if you are a vegetarian.
- Avoid consuming lots of sugar to prevent a heightened decrease in collagen production
- It might be tempting to soak in a hot bath during cold weather but you should keep that short to prevent skin dehydration and loss of natural body oils
- Get a humidifier to fill in for the loss of moisture the home heater sucks from the atmosphere
- Use your sunscreen as well. Just because it's winter does not mean that your screen should not be protected from UV rays. UV rays can cause damage to your skin at any time of the year so get your SPF on now.

Spring Skincare Secrets

As the weather changes from cool to warm, we must maintain healthy, radiant skin. Therefore, be prepared with your toner to brighten your skin after the season of drabness that winter brings. If you get any blemishes or dark spots throughout the winter, you should also treat your skin with serum or other treatments. Of course, no matter the season, your cleanser should always be nearby!

I'll step it up a notch in the following chapter with further advice on how to have healthy, glowing skin.

04

An Apple A Day

You've probably heard the proverb "an apple a day keeps the doctor away." It turns out that apples provide incredible nutrients that keep us healthy and powerful. Similarly, certain lifestyle recommendations maintain not just the health of our skin but also the health of our thoughts. In addition to using skin care products, there are several other things we may do to improve our health and wellness. Let me give you a personal example. One year, due to the demands of family life and my job, there was a time when I frequently was unable to follow my usual skincare routine. I instead ensured that I took my multivitamins and other health supplements. When I got some breathing room, I started my activities at the gym and had some tests done on my body to make sure I was healthy, which I was! My skin was healthy, my lungs were working properly, and my blood was pure. Impressed, my gym teacher advised me to keep doing whatever I was doing because it was benefiting me. I will discuss those details with you in this chapter.

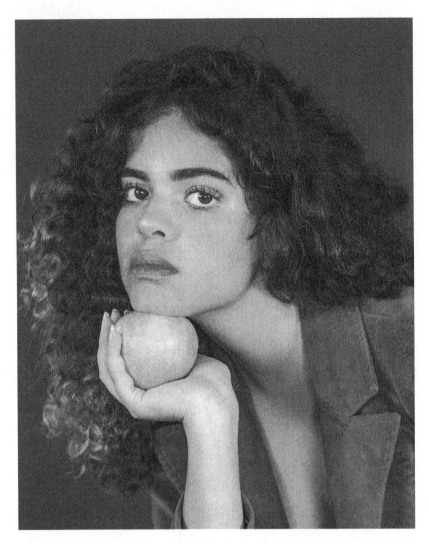

These are also lifestyle practices that, in my experience as a person of color, are absent from our communities. Although some of us already practice it, we still need more people to do so. For this reason, I urge you to inform as many people as you can to buy this book so that we can all stay healthy. Our bodies must be in good shape for us to fulfill our function on this planet. I'll give you my "apple-a-day" advice now without further ado. They are lifestyle advice, should we say.

Lifestyle Tips to Achieve Healthy and Glowing Skin

Be mindful of Your Physical Environment

Your skin can suffer negative effects from your environment.[15] Your skin has a lot to deal with, from sun exposure to the chill of winter to humid weather. Overexposure to the sun's UV radiation can destroy skin cells, which can lead to hyperpigmentation, wrinkles, rough skin, and, in the worst-case scenario, skin cancer.

In addition to sun exposure, extreme weather conditions can also harm our skin.

On the other hand, a little sun can do wonders for people of color, especially the Vitamin D-rich early morning rays. If you haven't already, make sure to read the chapter where I discussed how to care for your skin throughout the seasons.

Choose Your Social Environment

Your social circle affects how well you take care of your body. Do your friends care passionately about having beautiful skin? Although it may not be necessary for long-lasting friendships, there is nothing wrong with having your skin goals circle as part of your inner circle! Hahaha!

Drink a lot of Water

Yes, you are once again being told to drink water. Looking for a practical way to get beautiful, healthy skin? Get plenty of water. In addition to being healthy for your skin, it is also helpful for your

---

15   ("How do environmental factors affect our skin?" 2016)

general health. You risk becoming dehydrated and sustaining skin damage if your skin is dehydrated.

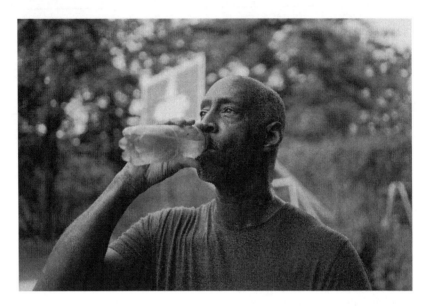

Here are some of the ways drinking water helps your skin:

- It helps to flush out toxins from your body thereby increasing your skin health. Some toxins clog your skin pores and cause acne, drinking water prevents such from happening.
- It helps to tighten your skin, especially after excessive weight loss which often leads to sagging skin. If you would like to tighten your skin, drink lots of water.
- It aids blood flow to the skin thereby improving your skin tone.
- It helps to maintain your skin's pH level. Clean water has a pH level of 7, hence its suitability for maintaining healthy skin.
- If you drink enough water, you are less likely to develop wrinkles, scars, and lines. As you get older, your body will

find it hard to retain water, so keep your body hydrated and refreshed.

- If you are regularly exposed to the sun, you should make drinking water a priority in your skincare routine.
- Do you often have a puffy face? That may be a sign that you aren't drinking enough water, so drink it more!
- If you have dry skin and don't drink enough water as well, you will be prone to itchy skin, flakiness, and cracks.
- In addition, bathing keeps your skin clean, unclogs pores, and moisturizes.

A typical adult needs at least 7 glasses of water each day, but your needs may vary based on your weight, height, metabolism, and daily activities. Consult your physician.

Skin Treatments

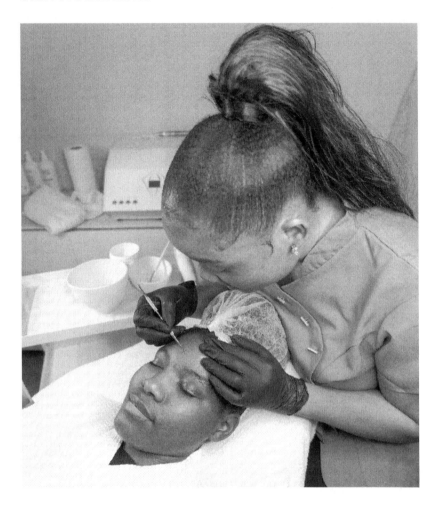

Skin care procedures were briefly mentioned in Chapter 2, and I'm bringing them up once more due to their significance. Treat any skin condition you develop—acne, fine wrinkles, keloids, etc.—before it worsens! Consult your skin care specialist if the situation doesn't improve.

Have a Skin Care Routine

One cannot overstate the value of a skincare regimen, especially for people with a darker complexion. Our well-being depends on the health of our skin. It shields us from diseases, bacteria, and infections. Even if your skin appears healthy, you cannot be certain of that unless you examine it carefully; however, with a regular skincare program, you can be certain of that.[16]

By

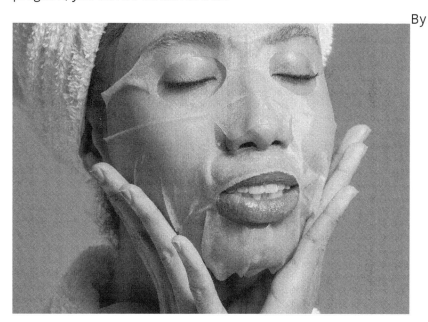

removing dead skin cells with a skincare program, new, healthy skin cells can grow. Go to the prior chapter for more information on the skincare regimen that will give you healthy, beautiful ebony skin.

Have Your Bath Twice A Day

It may go against your instinct to take a bath twice a day but do so. Even though your skin seems clean because of the frigid climate where you dwell, take a bath twice a day. Although bathing and skin

---

16   (Chukwuemeka 2021)

care are separate topics, it's vital to remember that they are very beneficial for your lovely ebony skin. For example, lukewarm water bathing not only clears clogged skin pores but also improves blood circulation.

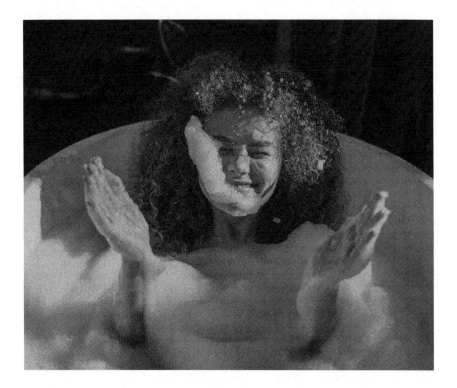

To remove any filth that might have accumulated throughout the day, I advise taking a bath twice a day: in the morning and at night. Dead skin cells are removed in this way by washing, and new ones are given space to come to life!

Exercising

Exercise is great for your skin, yet many people exercise only to reduce weight. It aids in enhancing circulation and blood flow, which in turn nourishes your cells. Healthier skin cells are the result of enhanced toxin elimination and improved blood flow! Stress has also been linked to poor skin health because it makes the body release hormones that can cause allergies, breakouts, and skin inflammation.

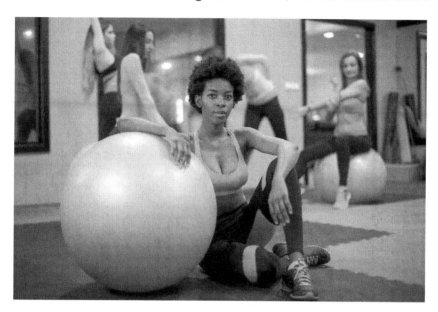

Exercise can help you fight skin-related problems by lowering your body's sensitivity to stress and boosting your immune system. While exercising, use sunscreen to protect your skin from the sun. Afterward, take a shower to remove sweat to avoid chafing and rashes. Ladies resist the urge to apply makeup while working out because it will simply clog your skin pores and lead to breakouts.

Multivitamins

I like multivitamins! You would notice that Vitamin D, Vitamin C, Vitamin A, and Vitamin E are frequently included as mainstay ingredients in the skin care products I suggested to you if you paid attention to the active ingredients list. Particularly if you live in a cold climate, you should consume vitamin D frequently. In Africa, we have the wonderful morning light to provide the vitamin D we require, but outside of Africa, things are different. We must find our source of vitamin D! Black people should take vitamin D supplements when going to Europe or other cold climates. However, for the correct dosage, check with your doctor.

Diet

Have you ever noticed how the sweetest things aren't always the healthiest? They're also bad for your skin. If you want to have healthy, glowing skin, avoid carbonated beverages. You can have them once in a while (like once in a blue moon), but don't make them a regular part of your diet. This is because sugar inhibits collagen production in your body, resulting in saggy skin. Although not directly related to diet, smoking is another habit you should avoid if you care about your skin's health. I know these two — sugar and smoking — are difficult to give up if addicted, but it is worth a shot.

Medical Checkup

Many skin conditions have been aggravated or caused by underlying health issues. If you notice any changes in the colour or texture of your skin or experience any itching for a protracted period, see your doctor!

Sleep

You should think about getting some beauty rest. The benefits of sleeping between seven and nine hours per night for your skin are numerous.

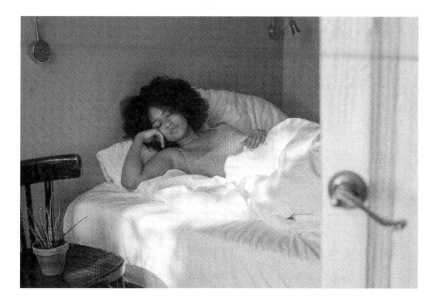

- Sleep allows your skin cells to regenerate and rebuild.
- It removes toxins and repairs skin cells that have been damaged by environmental factors such as sun exposure and pollution.
- It keeps the skin moisturised after a long day in the sun's ultraviolet rays.
- It promotes the production of collagen, which improves the elasticity of your skin.
- It increases blood flow, which transports nutrients to your skin.
- Sleep aids in the reduction of cortisol levels in the body. If you don't get enough sleep, your cortisol levels will remain elevated, leading to aging and possibly acne flare-ups!

The importance of sleep in maintaining healthy, glowing skin cannot be overstated. So pay attention to your sleep.

With this, we've reached the end of this lovely book, and I hope it's of great help to you on your skincare journey. However, I'd like to emphasize that the information in this book is not intended to guarantee results. It also does not establish any aesthetician-client relationship between us. So be cautious now. And, while I believe I did a good job of providing the resources you need to achieve healthy, glowing skin, this book is not a substitute for the advice of a dermatologist.

Finally, I look forward to hearing from you and answering your questions. On Instagram, you can find me at @embeautyaesthetics. Also, make sure to share this book with your family, friends, and anyone else who wants to learn how to care for their skin! That being said, take care of your beautiful black skin and keep an eye out for my social media posts. Take care!

References

1. "The Best Moisturizers for Your Skin Type." n.d. Dermstore. Accessed December 17, 2022. *https://www.dermstore.com/blog/best-moisturizers-dry-oily-sensitive-skin/.*

2. Chukwuemeka, Blessing. 2021. "Beauty hacks for the African Skin." Melange Africa. *https://www.melangeafrica.com/beauty-hacks-for-the-african-skin/.*

3. Cobb, Cynthia, Cammy Pedroja, and Sarika Ramachandran. 2020. "Sebum: What Is It, How to Remove Excess on Face, Hair, Scalp, More." Healthline. *https://www.healthline.com/health/beauty-skin-care/sebum.*

4. "Dry Skin." 2019. Harvard Health. *https://www.health.harvard.edu/a_to_z/dry-skin-a-to-z.*

5. "15 Best Moisturizers For Black Skin In 2022 (Face & Body)." 2022. The Chic Pursuit. *https://chicpursuit.com/best-moisturizers-for-black-skin/.*

6. "How do environmental factors affect our skin?" 2016. AP Skincare. *https://www.apskincare.co.uk/blog/how-do-environmental-factors-affect-our-skin/.*

7. Kimball, AB. n.d. "Comparison of the epidemiology of acne vulgaris among Caucasian, Asian, Continental Indian and African American women." PubMed. Accessed December 17, 2022. *https://pubmed.ncbi.nlm.nih.gov/21108671/.*

8. "Melasma: Causes." 2022. American Academy of Dermatology. *https://www.aad.org/public/diseases/a-z/melasma-causes.*

9. Mitchell, Amanda. n.d. "How to Choose the Right Facial Cleanser Dermstore." Dermstore. Accessed December 17, 2022. *https://www.dermstore.com/blog/different-types-of-cleansers/.*

10. Obafemi Awolowo University, Ladoke Akintola University of Technology, and Bolaji Otike-Odibi. 2019. "African Skin: Different Types, Needs, and Diseases." Research Gate. *https://www.researchgate.net/publication/333692639_African_Skin_Different_Types_Needs_and_Diseases.*

11. Oliveira, Marilyn. n.d. "What Is the Baumann Skin Type." Dermstore. Accessed December 17, 2022. *https://www.dermstore.com/blog/the-baumann-skin-type/*.

12. Ollennu, Amerley. 2021. "5 common skin concerns for Black men and what to do about them - Etre Vous." Etrevous. *https://www.etrevous.com/Blogs/Skincare/Advice/5-common-skin-concerns-for-black-men-and-what-to-do-about-them*.

13. Quinn, Jessie. n.d. "What Do Face Serums Do? We Find Out." Dermstore. Accessed December 17, 2022. *https://www.dermstore.com/blog/top_ten/what-are-face-serums/*.

14. Racho, Janeca. n.d. "Intro Guide to Product Types." Dermstore. Accessed December 17, 2022. *https://www.dermstore.com/blog/skin-care-101/*.

15. Rattan, Dr. V. 2022. *Skin Revolution: The Ultimate Guide to Beautiful and Healthy Skin of Colour*. N.p.: HarperCollins Publishers Limited.

16. Smith, K. R., and D. M. Thiboutot. 2008. "Thematic review series: Skin Lipids. Sebaceous gland lipids: friend or foe?" jlr.org. *http://www.jlr.org/content/49/2/271.full*.

17. Yowell, Hanna. n.d. "Are You Using The Right Routine For Your Skin Type?" Heyday. Accessed December 17, 2022. *https://www.heydayskincare.com/blogs/skin-deep/skin-type-v-skin-conditions*.

About the Author

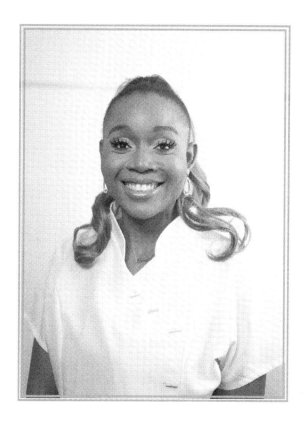

Emade Masango is an aesthetician who discovered her passion for skincare after having trouble with her skin during pregnancy. Since then, she has never stopped helping others with similar skin conditions by offering beauty services such as facials, skin treatments, manicures, pedicures, and more. Her goal is to empower black communities around the world one skin at a time. She is always laughing and curious, and she enjoys both lighthearted and serious conversations about skincare, health and wellness, personal development, and wealth creation in the black community. You can follow her on Instagram at @embeautyaesthetics!

Made in the USA
Columbia, SC
25 May 2023

16725450R00055